WAR ON MY BELLY
How to Work Out a Workout While Working

David Chen and Nora Mousas

ISBN: 978-0-9861612-0-9 (sc)
ISBN: 978-0-9861612-2-3 (hc)
ISBN: 978-0-9861612-1-6 (e)

Library of Congress Control Number: 2015904645

Because of the dynamic nature of the Internet, any web addresses or links contained in this book may have changed since publication and may no longer be valid. The views expressed in this work are solely those of the author and do not necessarily reflect the views of the publisher, and the publisher hereby disclaims any responsibility for them.

Any people depicted in stock imagery provided by Thinkstock are models, and such images are being used for illustrative purposes only. Certain stock imagery © Thinkstock.

Lulu Publishing Services rev. date: 4/6/2015

CONTENTS

ACKNOWLEDGMENTS

To my loving family who motivates me to get healthy, and to my employers and co-workers who allowed (and still allow) me to practice healthy working habits.

IN THE BEGINNING...

In the beginning, it came to the author's attention that it would be best to add some credence to his brand new book by introducing a central idea from Eastern healthcare practices. Thus, he brings to you the following Chinese proverb - the best doctors treat the perfectly healthy human beings:

Long, long ago, in a place and time you've probably never been to, the most famous surgeon in all the land was brought to the king. The king, you see, wanted to know how he had so quickly perfected his medical practice.

The surgeon was astonished by such praise, exclaiming that he was not even the best doctor in the area. "In fact," he told his king, "I would only rank myself as the third-best doctor in this land."

The king was, in turn, astonished by the surgeon's reply. "You're kidding me, right?! You're highly regarded all over this country. Who exists in this land that's a better doctor than you, and how come I've never heard of this person?"

"Well, I have an older brother," the surgeon replied. "His patients always get treated in the early stages of illness. Even so, he's still only the second-best doctor." He paused. "But in the end, I would have to say that our oldest brother really is the best doctor I've ever met. He has a list of patients who never get sick, because he cares for them before they even catch their disease. Then again," he continued, "it's natural that you've heard less of them and more about me."

The king, at this point suitably confused, attempted to interject but was quickly cut off as the surgeon (rather obliviously) continued.

"You hear about me because I cut people open and perform complicated surgeries. People talk about me because everyone likes hearing stories about people being sliced open, rearranged, and miraculously restored."

The king, being one of those people that enjoyed hearing about body parts and blood, agreed.

"If you think about it, though, this is proof that I don't do my job nearly as well as my brothers do. The only reason I need to perform all these complicated surgeries is because I'm not good at treating small symptoms before they become major problems, like my brothers do."

Thus the king, suitably wowed by this explanation, promptly beheaded the poor doctor and sought out his older brother in his place...

...Just kidding. The doctor was set free to pursue the next several decades of his life while his oldest brother was subsequently questioned by the king. Nevertheless, the proverb still adequately illustrates the main idea this book will try to teach you: the key to a cure might lie in treating yourself in your own living and working spaces before getting sick.

Prevention. Early detection. Treatment

These are things that could all be initiated by you with helps from those top rated people who specialize in healthcare. The most effective medical practitioners learn to treat people who are not yet patients, and those are the doctors you should talk to before getting ready for that long hospital stay and arguing with insurance companies. Good doctors stop small symptoms from turning into major diseases and know you like family, but probably won't be famous enough to be on TV or treat professional athletes. Then there are the normal and average doctors who are busy treating diseases.

Because of the existence of such a profit oriented ranking scale in the current medical system, it is difficult to find that caring doctor who gives you medical advice before you get sick. But--news flash--you don't necessarily have to find one. The secret to good health starts from (get ready for it) yourself! Living a lifestyle that prevents disease is the essence of best medical care. Plus, who else can better monitor the small changes happening inside you? Be vigilant in taking note of any small decline in health and keep putting in some maintenance work, like you would do around your house. After all, most people would agree that being healthy is a big, big part of life, liberty and the pursuit of happiness, if not the biggest part.

PROLOGUE

If you're my age, you've probably heard phrases like "War on Drugs" or even "War on Hollywood" littered around the media, political campaign speeches and (of course) the Internet. We spend a lot of time and energy focusing on big problems; social problems concerning other people and society as a whole, things we have little control over. But in reality, dealing with some of the "personal" problems we have closer to home would also help make the world a much better place. Usually, "me, me, me" or "my, my, my" is a selfish and non-effective attitude when dealing with social problems. But when it comes to weight problem, there is no urgent need to go "social". "War! What is it good for..."? Just look down on my middle section and I found at least one answer. It would have made a big difference in the world if more office folks realize this. Barring periods of revolution or great social upheaval, change happens--much like the way we control our belly fat--bit by bit, one willing and responsible individual at a time.

It's easy to notice the problems of others if they are on TV or in the news constantly. But without reminders, we tend to ignore problems happening to ourselves, even problems happening in our body and mind.

Problems like--oh, I don't know--belly fat?

Common wisdom keeps telling us: once the dreaded belly fat casts its spell on you, it's next to impossible to get rid of. When trying to change the shape of something (like, to take a completely random example, a bulging waistline), one method is to grab it violently and squeeze it into shape, like it's wronged your family. The problem with this approach, apart from the fact that most of us don't have a hand big enough to wrap around a big belly, is that the shape it's been changed into doesn't hold. It's always hard to mold a problematic object to your heart's desire in a short period of time...and yet, that's the way a lot of fitness practices introduced in the world are programmed. As soon as the pressure's off, the "achievements" gained in a lot of fitness practices will vaporize. People can cram in exercises like they're competing in a reality show, striving to become "the biggest loser," and then proceed to revert back once it's all over.

If you pour water over a rock, the rock erodes gradually over a very long period of time. This process is what causes landscapes like the Grand Canyon to form, and guarantees long-lasting and consistent change. I'm not saying that you should pour water on your belly for hundreds of years, of course (not sure you'd live that long). But I am speaking metaphorically--I'm saying that only adapting gradual changes and integrating them into your daily life can create a permanent effect.

The patient and balanced approach that I'm advocating involves constant adjustments from one state of equilibrium to the next, because that's the best way to produce a long lasting effect--moving slowly but surely towards the target weight and continuing to make progress. Is it possible to put spilled milk back in its container, or undo the cracks in your iPhone after you've dropped it on the ground a couple hundred times? I don't think so. Likewise, once you've molded your lifestyle into a series of healthy habits, it's not likely to go back to the old system.

A better metaphor is to think of a solid round pebble being ground into a smaller cylinder. Will it be possible to see that slimmed down cylindrical sculpture turning back into a spherical object again? We've just found the perfect way to become a "loser" and stay a "loser". Well actually, come to think of it, we want to be a loser but when reaching certain desired weight and getting to a certain fitness level, we don't want to be a "loser" forever. The term just have a bad ring to it, so just scratch that "stay a loser" part.

THE DEVIL IN THE DETAILS

Even after solidifying the role of patience in attacking weight problems, there are still other details to be worked out. A large portion of the various health and fitness tips floating around have one big problem--no matter how promising a workout routine looks, it's hard to find enough of that common yet precious thing called "time" to follow it. For us working class citizens, big portions of our day are often taken up by the cultural phenomenon widely known as "work". And no; even though "work" is the root word for "workout", they're about as different from each other as the difference between "water" and "water torture". Try as we might, we can't simply put on our swimsuits and go "one, two--take a step--three. four--looking good . . ." when it's 9 to 5 in the office. There are distinct possibilities of, y'know, getting caught and getting labeled as weird. In fact, one of the best case scenarios is just being called

1

crazy. The worst case scenario involves being sued and sent to a mental institution by employers and coworkers, needless to say, the job, reputation, and possibilities of future employment are lost. Working environments are just not as friendly towards laborious and backbreaking activities as it used to be like when we all worked in the fields.

Right... we didn't want to work too hard and wanted to get paid more, back when we were working in the fields. But it sure was healthier to one's body when moving around a lot. What if we can combine the good of both worlds of "field" and "desk" jobs? Who created this concept of "desk job" anyway? Can we get the "desk job" kind of pay, but still get "field job" amount of exercise daily?

In all seriousness, the standard office job just doesn't provide us with great opportunities to exercise any more. There was once a time where any job was synonymous with physical labor, but that system ended. With the arrival of new technology, we've replaced hours of tough physical exercise with...well, with hours of tough *mental* exercise. And no, those two don't really mean the same thing.

Even after office hours, there's a high chance that you're exhausted (just because physical and mental exercise aren't the same doesn't mean you can't feel the same way afterwards) and are reluctant to part way with that hard-earned paycheck to get to a gym. After all, memberships to the gym don't come cheap. And even *then*, if you manage to drag yourself to the gym and coerce yourself into getting a membership under heavy self-pressure, you're still faced with the reality that a second at the gym is a second that isn't being spent relaxing with your family, relaxing with your friends, relaxing with your cat or dog, or just relaxing in general. With this knowledge in mind, the membership wastes away in your wallet while you're off playing Yahtzee with your kids and we're back at square one.

Life is all about facing tough choices, dealing with dilemmas, and moving forward. It's that kind of thing that gave us desk jobs over fieldwork in the first place. With my own personal dilemma in mind, I've developed a way to combine my daily work with daily work*outs*. That way, I won't feel guilty for not working out even if I skip the occasional evenings at the gym...

Now, I'm going to whisper to you my secret system of getting a workout while you're in the office without getting your boss or co-workers annoyed, also without any degradation in your performance and productivity. It's pretty obvious that a light workout in a limited space is still, after all, a workout -- it can erode that belly fat away bit by bit. As I've stated before, those gradually removed pounds won't come back if you develop the habit; in this way, those office workout routines are actually good for you. They're lifestyle changes – type of changes growing into habit -- and are therefore more reliable than those sudden workouts and fads.

On the days I do visit gym, I only spend a small amount of time before going home, comfortable in the knowledge that I've been exercising the entire week. My gym membership isn't wasted, but I still get the luxury of free time to spend with my family.

THE CONSPIRACY

As a wise philosopher once said, people despise other people who make resolutions. And as an even wiser philosopher said, people despise others even more when those who make resolutions face-plant themselves, fail to make good on promises and change the status quo.

While I may not have actually taken these quotes from any philosopher, it's the unfortunate truth of human nature -- people take pleasure from observing other people's failures. The Germans even have a word for it: "schadenfreude".

In a similar way, I get the feeling telling my employers I intend to work out anywhere from three to six hours a day during working hours, before even starting, isn't exactly the best of ideas. At best, they'd sternly rebuke me. At worst, they'd wonder about the amount of ROI they were getting out of their investment in me (a.k.a. my paycheck). Instead, I decided to keep it a secret and just quietly doing my part to cut down the rising health care and insurance cost for the nation. No one can detect that I am not aligning my career goal along with the corporate objectives of my employer if I don't utter a word. But if I do mention anything at all, the sad thing is that even though I'm still producing the exact same quality and amount of work as before, many people would likely nod their heads and say: "yeah, he's a slacker" "he doesn't give 120% pulling his weight", just because I'm exercising absentmindedly while working.

See folks, obesity is in fact an occupational hazard for office workers nationwide, and reducing sick days out of my life long career is a noble cause for the society and all the nice folks around me. With this conspiracy in mind, I felt like I'm contributing tremendously to the company for which I work for and creating a lot of values for the shareholders. Wow, at this stage of my career, I have just reached a new level of excellence, and discovered the meaning of my existence!

When one has a noble aspiration as far-reaching as for the entire corporation, it is better not to say anything to co-workers, until that goal is reached and some tangible results are clearly attained. Eventually I would tell my co-workers and HR about how I've saved healthcare costs for the nation and for the society as a whole. Hopefully they would be able to appreciate how much savings coming back from the society and would feel the positive effects on all of us - the nice office mates surrounding me. I have fond memories of a TV commercial portraying an Italian immigrant who was a pizza entrepreneur. The little boy was dreaming about pizza in classroom and got misunderstood and got yelled at by his teacher, while simultaneously getting taunted by other classmates. In the final scene, he was expelled from school and stood on the top of a hill overlooking the school yard of his former alma mater. He announced loudly to the heaven and earth with a heavy Mediterranean accent: "one day, the entire world will thunk (sic) me".

BMI

Even though disease prevention is a noble cause, there's no money in it because it's hard for people to automatically notice and quantify its effects and benefits. Despite the fact that mankind as a general rule has better foresight than animals, most of us still cannot predict like the prophets of lore. I'm sure you yourself know a couple of people who cry "headache" when asked to think a bit further down the road. And if you don't know any people like that, then you are that person.

There's a story that goes something like this: a woman wanted to persuade her husband to quit smoking. Every time her husband bought cigarettes, she stashed away the same amount of money he spent. At the end of the year, she showed her husband how much money she'd saved, which was a measurement of how much he had lit away in smokes. With real money in front of his eyes, the husband was shocked at how much he'd consumed and decided to quit. He was able to stay clear from cigarettes for one year and, at the end of the following year, demanded the woman to show him the money saved. The woman couldn't show the husband the money because the savings had been spent along the way. Predictably, the "facts-and-figures" result-oriented husband went right back to smoking again.

How do we measure the amount of disease we've warded off by staying fit? It would be hard, if not impossible, to get an accurate measurement. If people knew the amount, would they change? How do we fix a problem that comes from avoiding exercise and eating too much, when society closes its eyes to it?

It's time for a pop quiz, everybody! Which type of mathematical study could help people discipline themselves more effectively?

A. Geometric shapes and forms: Push everyone to match up to impossible beauty standards.

In this appearance obsessed society, we *could* use peer pressure to shame people into starving themselves to death if they don't have a skinny body. Since peer pressure has already done so much damage to our society, it's about time that we finally use its positive side-effects to let everybody know beauty is really only skin deep, when it comes to belly fat. But in the meantime, the deep thoughts oriented crowed will argue inner beauty is more important and can make you happier, healthier and more successful, etc. We are going round and round in circles again, and that is why large amount of people keep going back to stuffing themselves to their big-belly-hood.

Nevertheless, considering mass media and a good number of crowd-minded teenagers do enough damage with this tactic already and we are still having an obesity epidemic on our hands. We've got people in schools, in offices, in pretty much every imaginable place we can think of murmuring to fat people why they don't "work out more" or "eat less". Considering the old saying that we shouldn't try failed methods "again and again", I think we can all agree that this isn't the way to go. In fact, it's pretty much the *opposite* of the way to go if only for the reason of political correctness--and ironically, it's kind of what's currently happening. Political correctness has the same effect as pressure packed gossips, words without a shred of action to reduce even one ounce of weight out of anybody.

B. Numbers: Find a numeric system that can accurately measure what's considered a healthy weight in comparison to your body type, and statistically measure and certify the correlation between happiness and those new body types.

Without quantitative standards, it's hard to be scientific. Without being scientific, it's hard to get this weight loss thing into a science. Luckily, there's an easily measurable parameter called BMI (body mass index) which is tightly related to one's health care spending and health status (and therefore by varying degrees of extension: mood, positive attitude, happiness, social presentability, self-esteem, confidence, appearance, WOW factors during job interviews and sales presentation swagger, and many, many other magical words and things). Oh, and did I mention how easily BMI is measured? For the most basic measurements, all you need to know is your weight and height; you can get a BMI value by dividing the two. After getting your BMI, you can use your favorite search engine such as Google to find the range of BMI values that is considered "healthy" for you.

(Oh, and for those of you who were wondering, the right answer was B.)

Since measuring BMI is so easy, it's the ruler by which we'll decide whether or not we've attained our goals of healthiness and happiness. From there, we can walk around with healthy BMI along with great attitude to convince people that staying fit is something measurable and worth doing. At a minimum, we can just be happy and pain free, presenting a big smile to or winking at ourselves.

Another nice thing about BMI is that it can be used to dissuade people from trying to lose weight for the sake of losing weight. After all, a healthy BMI has a range of values. When one's BMI is in the lower end of the appropriate range, it would be unhealthy to lose weight further. Furthermore, as we've established earlier, losing weight is a slow and steady progression. In the process of achieving a healthy BMI, one should pay close attention to themselves and make sure to take a step back if they're feeling nauseated, dizzy, or otherwise unwell. As long as you set your sights on a healthy BMI, health and fitness (happiness as a certain by-product) will surely come much like the sun rises after night. There's no point in torturing yourself to be "slim and skinny" or going after immediate results. The ultimate goal is to be happy and healthy, not to lose weight endlessly or starve yourself to death.

Fabricated statistics show that the healthy BMIs of a group of employees (and therefore the health of a group of employees) help the employers too. Ladies and gentlemen, Exhibit A: Myself. I know two facts about myself (aside from other things like my favorite color, birthday, and what I had for breakfast today): first, that my performance review at work (and therefore my paycheck) haven't been negatively affected. Second, I haven't asked for a sick day in years.

...On the other hand, I might've jinxed myself with that "second" point and contract the worst flu in the history of the world tomorrow, prompting me to take ten sick days in a row. Knock, knock on desk.

By looking at family history, I don't have very good genes to begin with and will most likely not live to break any world records for longevity. But I was born in a developing country and didn't have enough to eat while growing up. Even now, food is always precious to me. I could think of many ways to die that would be acceptable albeit odd, but dying of too much food would be the ultimate tragedy (and irony) for me. Thinking back on the hunger pangs I endured from numerous foodless nights in my youth, I can't allow my tombstone to be carved with the words:

"Here lies a chap who had a flat and at times even concave belly for the majority of his life. Sadly, after realizing the American dream and living in a country with no worry of food shortage, gluttony got the better of him and he eventually died of food overdose at a lifespan decades shorter than that he could have lived."

For one this would legitimately be a sad reason to die. In addition, I'm not sure all that would fit on a gravestone.

THE WILL

Boy! It's really *hard* not to get overweight in an office environment today. Looking around, I see a lot of bulging waistlines among all my co-workers. Obesity can cause a lot of long-term problems, especially down the road, that are often very serious and very difficult to pronounce. Just Googling terms like: "health problems associated with obesity" will present you with a list that spans multiple pages with page numbers neatly printed at the bottom of the screen.

Further research on any one of those items on the list is enough to scare me to death--quite literally. For example, take diabetes. Diabetes is a condition that can be dealt with through careful monitoring and insulin injections, yes, but you can't get rid of it completely. "Diabetes 'kinda' problem, comes with a lot of inconveniences that follow you for a lifetime, the rest of the way, until money or time runs out on you", some victims told me. Their advice to me was to stay away from it as early as I could detect any ominous signs, or I would carry a lot of regrets and guilt. Guilt? That's really frightening.

If I could reduce my chance of these diseases, I would. I often hear people talking about the KISS principle. Let's quote someone German again about the nature of war in general (yes, including the war on belly): "In war, everything is simple, yet the simplest thing is difficult."

By the way, that "someone" happens to be not just any German, the quote came from the war master himself-- the famous von Clausewitz.

The simple weight loss equation boils down to "calories in" vs. "calories out"; "eat less food" vs. "consume more energy"; "sit less" vs. "move more" and so on and so forth. After carefully thinking over these many pairs of "give" and "take", it seems like a pretty simple thing to lose weight, right? The most important thing, though ("the simplest thing is difficult," remember?), is to have the will to carry out a plan that complies with that thinking of contrasting pairs of actions.

What to eat, where to live, when to get up, what fitness equipment to use, whether to eat a bran diet, and things with weird names like "chi-chi berries"--there are a lot of things to consider when it comes to weight loss, but the important thing is that we're not tricked into gaining more calories than losing them. As far as weight loss goes, calorie accumulation is bad and calorie draining is good. It's as simple as that.

Some people say that genes have a lot to do with being overweight. Some co-workers have asked me if I've ever seen a fat or overweight Asian. That kind of remark borders on racism, if you ask me, because China is now ranked as the country with the world's second most severe obesity problem (by overweight population) and the ranking happens to match that of their economic ranking. People from any race can stuff themselves to death if they don't play it carefully with wealth. Looking at the participants in hot dog eating competitions, and it's not hard to notice the champions and contestants can come from any ethnicity. I have to confess that I once gained eight pounds after a week of hometown visit, eating all my favorite childhood foods. There's also another time I gained ten pounds in a week after changing jobs because I had to walk twenty minutes from the bus stop every day to a downtown high-rise for my old job, then I only had to park my car and step into a suburban five-story building for the new one. Thus, the obesity problem eventually still comes down to calories accumulated vs. lost. Genes have a little to do with it, but not to the point of determining anyone's ultimate fate on the scale.

If you have the will to cut down your weight and don't mind changing your lifestyle to include a lot of standing and walking every day, you'll find that starting and sustaining weight loss are easier than you think.

I'll only outline the basic framework to go through here, but you're welcome to adjust the plan when it comes to practicing the techniques I've mentioned. Since everyone knows their own body best, changing the execution slightly according to your body to facilitate your gradual lifestyle change doesn't hurt. The important thing is to maintain the will in the long run and not to torture yourself or get totally discouraged halfway.

MAIN PLOT

STANDING, WALKING, BELT-TIGHTENING

I stand or walk while I work about three to six hours a day. Human beings were never creatures designed to sit around all day (or even the majority of the day, for that matter). I myself grew up in an agrarian society, and it was rare to see people working in the fields sporting big bellies. It's completely different when working with a desk job. I have an office job now, of course, and I can feel that belly trying to bulge up like "flubber" in the movie with that name.

CHAIR

It might be counter-intuitive, but believe it or not, sitting puts more pressure on the spine than standing. Throughout the course of human history, we've been used to standing up more than we've been used to sitting down. As humanity progressed, people started finding faster modes of transportation--and even then, carriages and animals demanded out of riders, more leg work and balancing acts, than the modern cars. In short, our ancestors burned a lot more fat in their daily lives than we do nowadays.

Sometimes, I hear people talking about the two problems brought about by modern technology--obesity and eye problems. It wasn't uncommon to hear kids being called "four-eyes" in my old school for wearing glasses, because they stood out. Similarly, back in the day, people in my high school would bully kids who stood out in the weight department by calling them "chubby", because it was so rare to see a kid growing so much in that time. Nowadays, "slim" might as well be a nickname in the workplace for someone who works in an office and still maintains the kind of body outline he or she used to have, in high school or even in college.

The eye sight is nearly impossible to fix after the damage is done (without using some sort of still debatable surgery), but weight problems can be dealt with regardless of how old we are. Even so, it does become harder to change as time goes on. For me, the first course of action was to stand up and turn my "desk" job into a "field" job, preferably without reducing the size of my paycheck. That is another ironic thing isn't it? Why should we go through the educations and training, strive to get paid more, only to suffer the accumulation of fat around the waist? Who invented desks and didn't think about the consequences and associated working environmental hazard that came with it? Well, all those inventions were probably done pre-industrial revolution and who would have thought there could be a day when a significant portion of a nation would be sitting around all day, even if people get paid more and seem more productive. Such is the reality in a developed industrialized society, with practically no concerns for starvation.

To accomplish that desk-to-field job conversion, I started off by putting my chair in the center of my cubicle and walking around it whenever possible. Thanks to my employer and his penchant for cordless telephones, I can easily walk around when making or answering calls. It's a small thing, sure, but I've noticed that most other people in the office sit while using those devices even though they *could* take advantage of the untangled and liberating wireless options. Well, that chair sure is addicting. In the end, however, standing and walking helped me feel more relieved and pressure-free. That chair was addicting to me just like to others, but eventually standing can become addicting too.

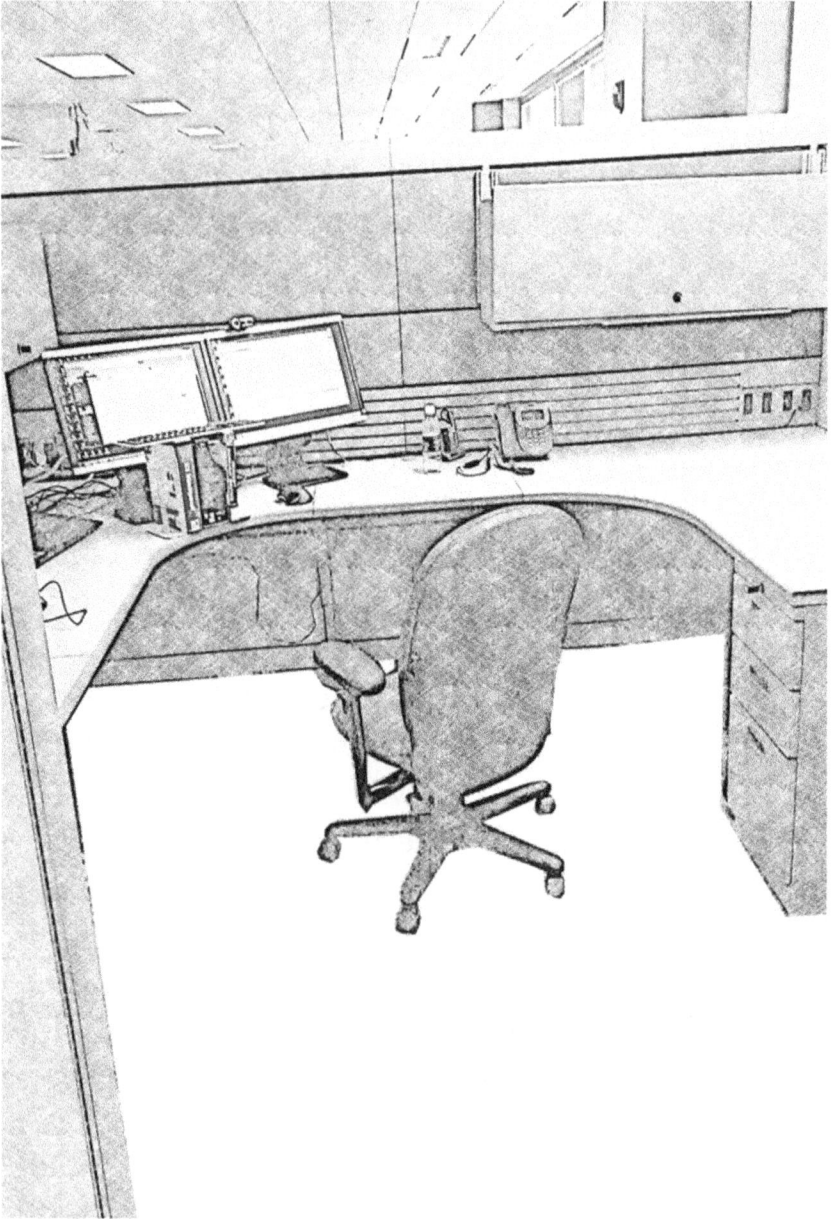

(This is how I see my office during a long day)

After standing and walking more, I started thinking that our attachments to desks and chairs aren't good for health in the office, yet we keep on attaching. We call our phones "desk phone", our job "desk job" and our leaders "chair persons". Let's see how smart leaders detached themselves from desks and chairs. I once had a boss who made a habit of walking to people whenever he needed to talk to someone in the same office location, conversing face to face instead of using the phone. That way, he could fit in a bit of walking in addition to being touted as a "people person."- What a deal! Of course (to the point of this book--shocking!) he wasn't overweight at all. That's what I call seniority and savvy professionalism. Kids, take notes.

By imitating him, I found that walking around in the office can help office employees gain a myriad of benefits, such as pulling oneself out of the foul mood when the office happens to have added many new aesthetically designed furniture, or purchased some ergonomically constructed interesting equipment, or happened to have some scenic surrounding along the walking routes. If one seeks to get humor out of the mundane and ordinary office work and to relieve the stress associated with the routines, what better way are out there than overhearing colleagues talking about each other behind their backs? I believe that's how movies, TV shows, and literary products like "Office Space" were inspired, but can't confirm.

The best way to catch office gossip is by walking around and keeping your eyes and ears wide open. If you happen to overhear people talking about you behind your back -- that will really make your day. But unfortunately, the chances of hearing other people talking about you randomly are slim, so you have to settle for a much more common occurrence of overhearing gossips about other people. Still, the entertainment value of office conversations is not to be underestimated. Keep cool, be a good office citizen, smile and wave. More importantly, don't spread any rumors.

Once in a while, when you go to another floor while trying to locate a colleague, try taking a small detour so you can walk a little more. For instance, if you get off the elevator knowing he or she is just about 20 feet away from the elevator by one route and 200 feet away by another, take the longer trail. Trust me, your productivity won't suffer *and* you'll get to know more people in the office, building your network and bridges and be "liked" by more people in the corporate social media on the intranet; it's really a win-win.

(It's a Choose-Your-Own-Adventure story.)

If anyone has any doubts about your productivity, go to the last section of this book and find the GDP calculation equations to support your argument.

Unfortunately, my work doesn't heavily consist of tasks that require verbal communication. I don't very often have meetings, teleconferences, presentations or classroom training sessions like some of my other co-workers. Otherwise, I would've had a field day (pun intended) with this part of my routine. I'm a programmer doubled as a professional email writer (or a "coder", as they like to call it). When I'm not having some sort of conversation (whether over the phone or in person), I'm most likely typing something with a computer keyboard in front of me. When typing, who's to say I can't stand by my table while doing so? I try to distant my buttocks from that thing called a "chair" as much as possible, at least in part because I've just learned a new word called "coccydynia" from a few fellow workers with job descriptions similar to mine.

The word itself doesn't sound good to me, whatever it means. Feeling the office chairs seem to hold some sort of black magic, I was determined to treat my office chair like I treat picnic chairs along the hiking trails in the park; unless I'm really, *really* tired, I'm not going to sit on them.

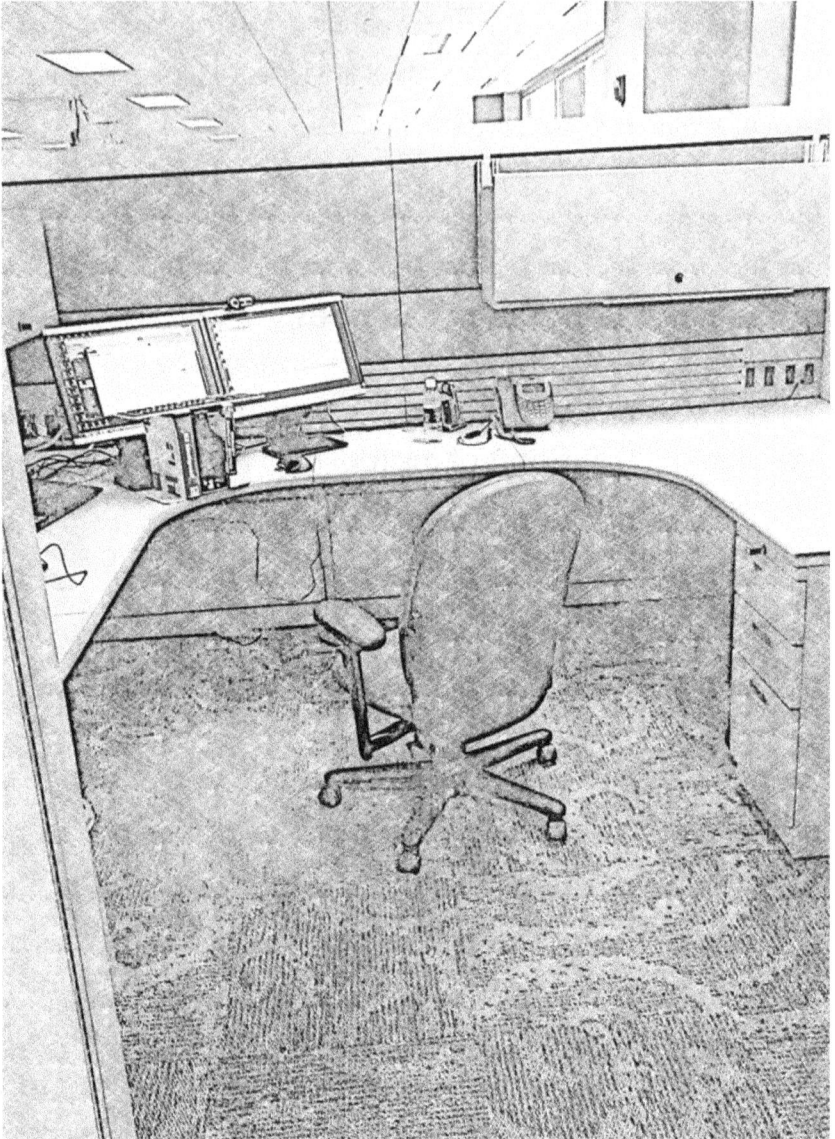

(Caution: Sitting on this chair will result in mental self-criticism.)

When I'm not putting the chair in the center of my cubicle, I'll shove it into the corner to give myself more room to walk. I like to walk in repeated paths--for example, an "8" shaped path, or a zigzag.

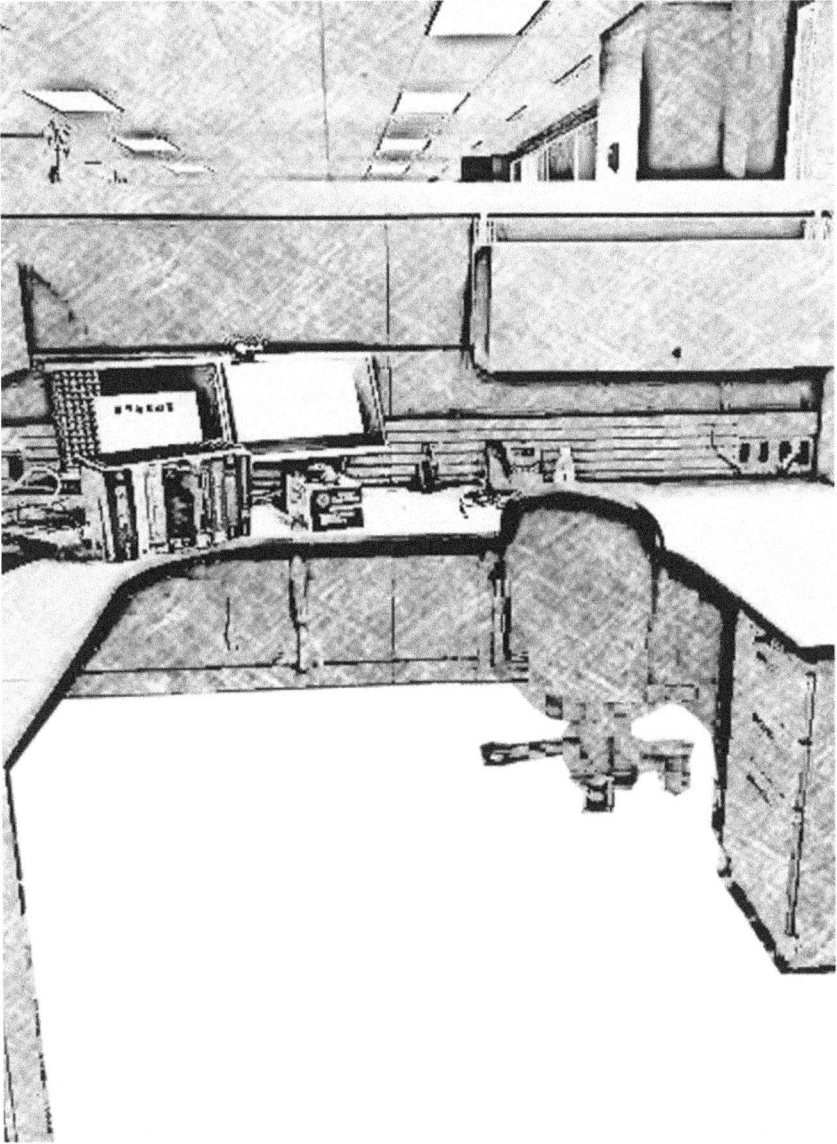

(It's like Columbus exploring the New World.)

KEYBOARD AND MONITORS

Since I didn't want to raise too much of a fuss about my fitness routine or cause any unnecessary trouble, I didn't go to HR to ask for a standup desk.

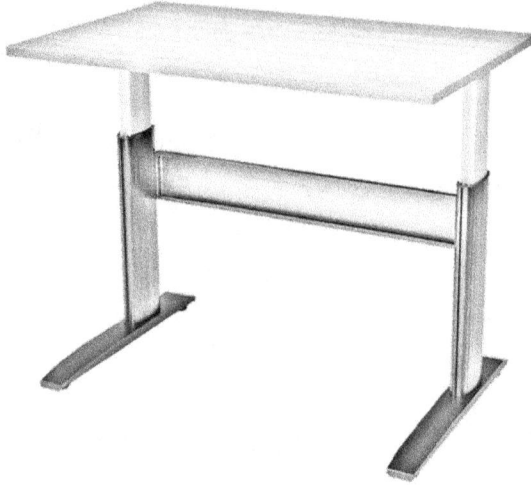

I didn't ask for converters that could turn my table into a standup setting, either.

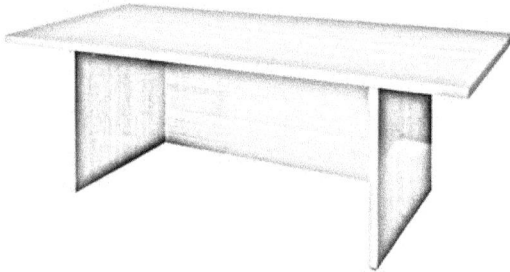

Our company policy stands like this: for employees with doctor's notes, HR can accommodate and make special arrangements for "timely" orders of standup desks or conversion stands. Since I don't have a doctor's note, I can't get a standing desk. Naturally, I decided to pass that opportunity to get a standing arrangement through HR so I can avoid getting a doctor's note, and be "timely" on my schedule of preemptive strike in this war on belly.

One other bad thing about the permanent standup setting is: what happens when one wants to sit down occasionally. Would you have to stop working? It is actually better to have the flexibility of being able to alternate easily between the two sets of arrangements, standing up and sitting down.

Among fitness fanatics, there's the occasional *fanatic* suggestion of installing a treadmill with a stand-up table in the office. To that approach, I would recommend moderation. The problem with a "live and kicking" treadmill is that such a machine has its own mind. Once the speed and inclination settings are punched in, it'll stubbornly insist that you keep walking in that certain way. If you're not careful, a treadmill in the office can transform into that famous 1958 Plymouth Fury called "Christine" huffing and puffing with furious engine noises, while demanding respect, as in the movie of the same name. How you envision what happens next is up to you, but let's just say it's not pretty.

Realistically, until the day comes when you can use brainwaves to control and change the values of pace and inclination for the treadmill, you won't be able to multitask and get any real work done on a treadmill. Again, we're talking about how to get a workout while doing some real work; in comparison, using a treadmill would probably either end with less work getting done or the type of slip and fall that ends up on "AFV." I've found that the people who can even get a treadmill installed at workplace are usually self-employed, employees working from home, or people with big enough corner offices. In those cases, they can go "one, two--take a step--three, four--looking good. . ." all day if they want to, and there wouldn't be any need for them to buy this book.

We're recommending a reasonable and low-profile approach to fitness, so it's probably best not to create big distractions in the office. A treadmill just isn't suitable enough for office use. If you want the changes to stick, you need to ease them in and make sure they're reasonable. It's one thing to be called "unique" or "different", and it's an entirely different thing altogether to be called "weird" or "insane".

After searching far and wide, I deduced that the best way to work out without losing productivity is by grabbing some old books and using a stack of them as a stand. After you place your keyboard on top, it functions as the perfect tool to get you to your feet. From there, forming another stand for the mouse is even easier than forming one for the keyboard.

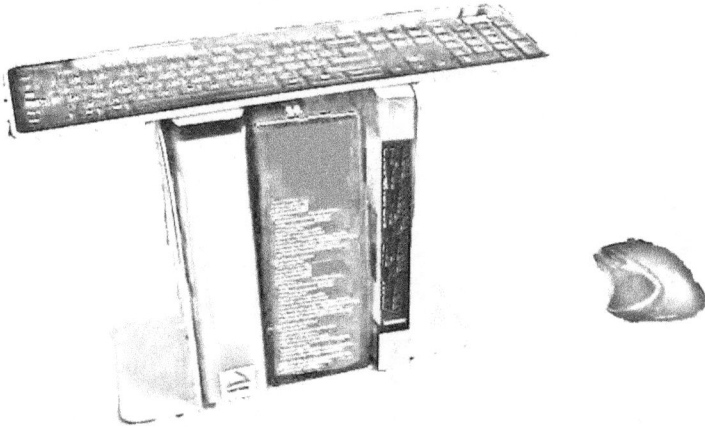

(I call this the "Leaning Tower of Technology".)

As for the monitors, I was pleasantly surprised to find that almost all of the flat panel monitors could be tilted upwards and seen while standing up. Maybe the monitor manufacturers had anticipated that there would be office workers like me, who would get tired of sitting and typing all day and try standing and typing instead. Or maybe they just wanted to advertise a higher range of motion, or could it be more to this? Is this a sign from the divinity calling for "standians" to accompany the "vegetarians" in the history of health and fitness training? The world may never know.

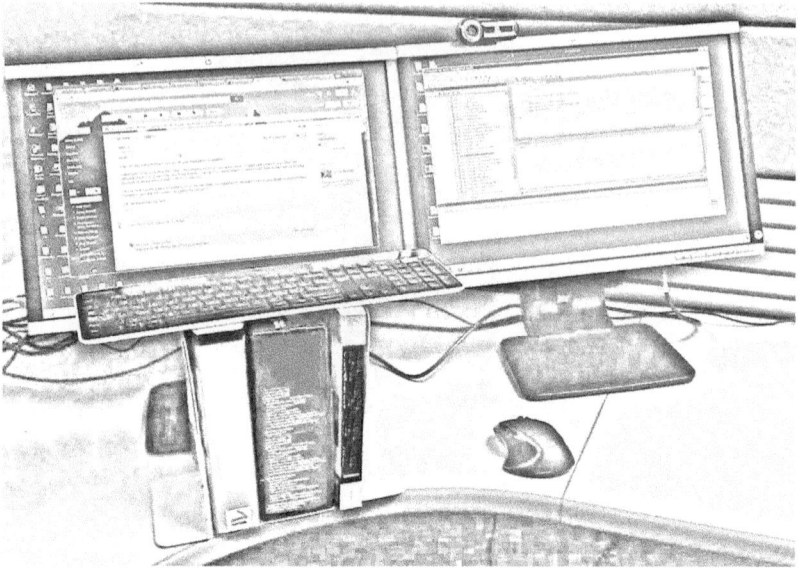

(I took this one from Leonardo da Vinci's sketchbook.)

WALKING

My favorite Bruce Lee quote is "be water, my friend." Usually, the limited space in a cubicle makes it difficult to walk in. This problem is easily solved by pretending I'm cooler than I really am and by walking in irregular and narrow zigzag lines like a Tai Chi master. In fact, it's even better for your health than walking in straight lines all day. There are TV programs demonstrating how to do Tai Chi in trans-Pacific flights, and the fact that we haven't (yet) heard of any in-flight fistfights triggered by this, or fight club planes just goes to show you how limited a space you need to practice workout and exercise your limbs. Walking in irregular directions slowly can exercise different muscle groups that you don't often use, which are silently aging and weakening within you.

No, those slow-motioned Tai Chi moves can't beat up anybody. That's not the point of them. Like many others kids of my age, I've wondered before about why Tai Chi is different from other forms of martial arts too. The slow motions of Tai Chi are for exercising and relaxation, even though the fast motions (any kind of fast moves, really) that can kick somebody's rear do exist. We're not going to talk about Tai Chi as a fighting technique but instead as a stretching and calming technique for our body and mind.

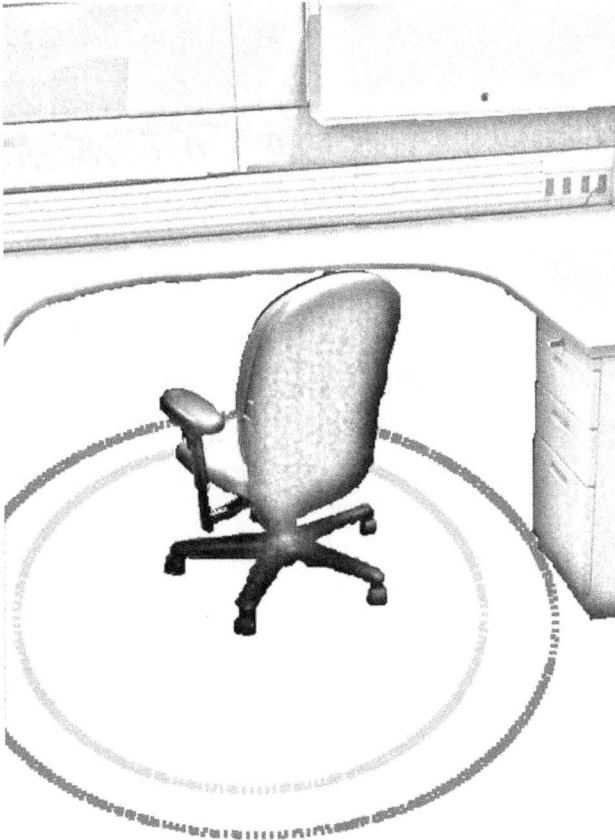

(Untested Scientific Theory:
An office chair lies in the center of the galaxy)

Now that we're not sitting in that office chair, we can walk around it. When you're tired, you can have a water break and sit on it as if you're in a park and walking on a hiking trail. The difference is that you're in an office, not a park. Try and walk when you're thinking and talking, and use the chair as little as possible.

Dehydration is a bad idea no matter whether you're exercising in a park or in an office, so it's important to drink plenty of fluids. With the new increase in your amount of daily exercise, you'll find that you might get dehydrated or dizzy, more easily. If that happens, you obviously wouldn't be able to properly continue exercising or focusing on work. In fact, you might even lose interest in exercising and derail the entire plan. We don't want to make those New Year resolutions and then give up and make the same New Year resolution again next year, so we should avoid getting dehydrated. The key to the entire experience is to keep it as pleasant and effective as possible, so know when to endure and when to sit down and take a breather.

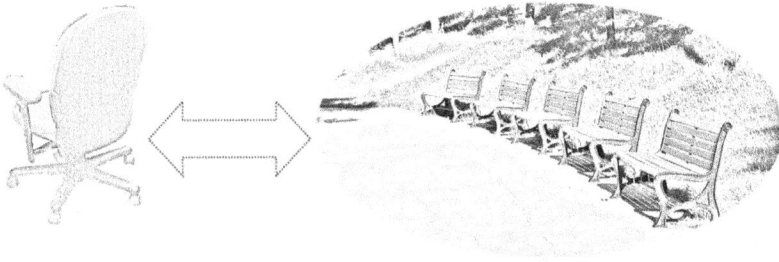

(Although maybe you shouldn't take your office
chair to the park with you.)

After walking around your chair for a while and getting your co-workers used to the idea that you like to stand while working, you're probably ready to start walking in an expanded area. You can start and give yourself more space by pushing the chair to the corner, and venture into the hall way occasionally; this enables you to walk more continuously without pausing or turning to change directions. You'll soon find that there are many patterns to walk in--straight lines, curved lines, zigzags, random shapes, you name it. Some of your coworkers might even follow in your footsteps and start to walk more themselves, one, two, three, we are now working on getting the fourth guy. As you know the term "guys" in office includes male and female . . . .

If you're lucky enough to have a corner office, you'll have much more space to walk in. In addition, your pedometer reading will probably present a more accurate representation than that of one in a smaller cubicle. A more accurate recording can usually give you a sense of accomplishment and more enthusiasm.

If you happen to be on the lower level of the food chain (like me), you might only be able to walk about three small steps along each side of the cubicle. Even so, there are still ways to develop a complex walking pattern. The important thing is to stay upright or in motion as long as possible.

If you put a chair in the middle of your office and just run circles around it, your head will probably start spinning within the space of seconds due to the same constant and inert motion pushing inside your brain. To save yourself from monotony, it's best to switch around the patterns you use. There are also certain patterns that can help you make the most of your limited space; for example, take the tango pattern below. The trick is to avoid disturbing others by walking slowly and gently. No matter how excited you are, it's probably not a good idea to disturb your co-workers by dancing loudly in the office (unless you've just gotten a big promotion). Try taking a step every couple of seconds; that way, the people that glare at you over their cubicle walls every ten minutes will get bored (preferably sometime before five sideway glances and not, y'know, five hundred). The most likely scenario is that your co-workers will simply get used to your new habit and turn their attention to other, more important things.

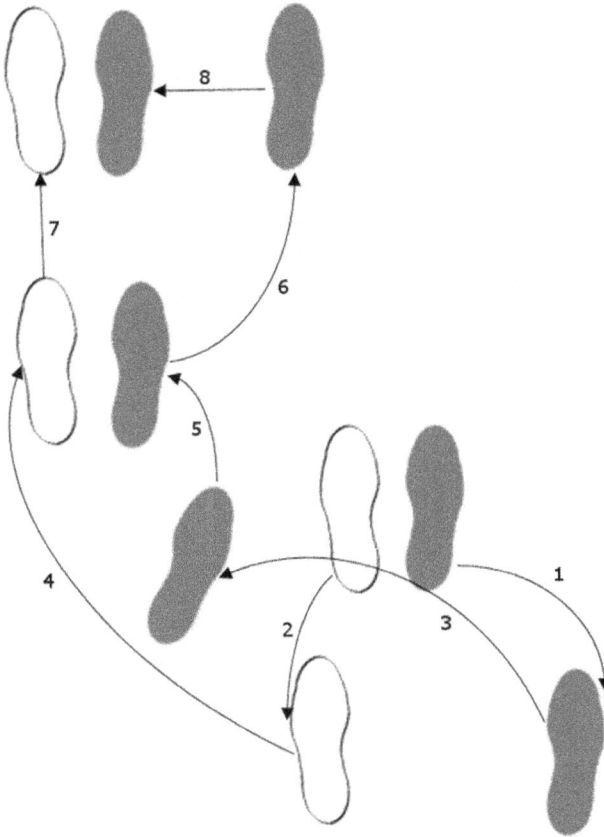

(I call this one the "Ten-to-Five Tango". It's a hit at the club.)

If you feel that your dancing steps aren't ideal for your cubicle, or that following the pattern will distract you from your work, you can simply walk backward. If you'd prefer to do this without colliding with (insert quite literally any and all objects in your particular office here), you can check the technique below.

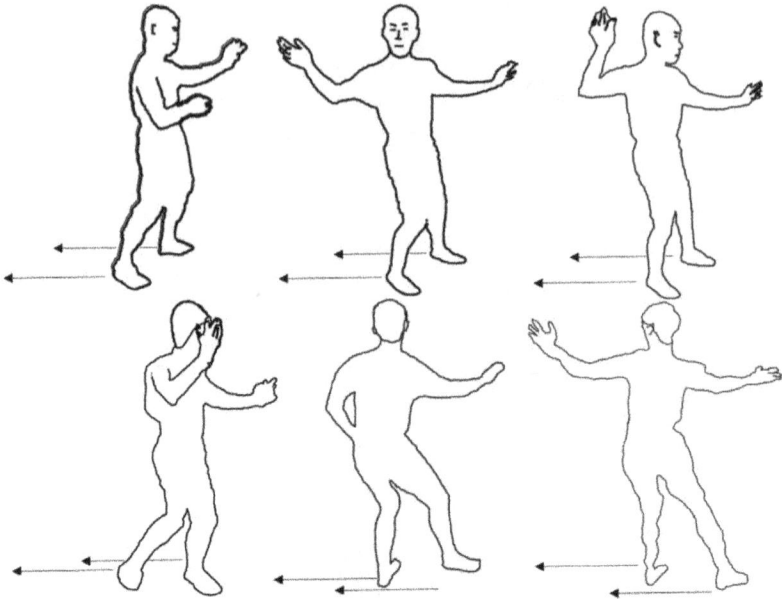

(Do you like the diagram? I drew it myself.)

Simply swivel your head from left to right, letting your arms follow along while walking backwards. Once you've managed to practice the motions enough to execute them smoothly (you'll realize, it doesn't take long), you can do it while talking on the phone to others. Just remember not to *actually* wave your hands back and forth like the little figures in the illustration; it's a surefire way to either get your fingers cracked on some office furniture or get HR sending someone to visit you. The technique is designed to help you simulating how to grow a pair of eyes at the back of your head, to avoid bumping into things while you're walking backward. After you've started, just concentrate on footwork for your office exercise.

Even with the dramatic arm swinging motion hidden, walking backwards in that way helps you exercise your neck muscles alongside helping you, not get injured. The motion can also help you get rid of your stiff shoulders if you throw your shoulders round and round slightly.

When you've had enough exercise, remember to take a seat and have a break. Don't be too aggressive and accidentally twist your neck or burn yourself out in the beginning. After all, the war on belly is at least a long term war, try "seven year war", if not a "thirty year war" or a "hundred year war". Not sure how many people can live that long for this last one, but the point is don't try to be a hero or a casualty too soon, at least try not to get hospitalized too soon. If you can't persist and persevere to fight another day, there will be no victory. A "battle of bulge" is not going to cut it--a "battle" is for the short term, and you need to treat the fight for your health as a "war."

To find a quantifiable way to measure how much we're exercising, you might want to consider getting a pedometer. A pedometer is a wonderful and mysterious device invented by a wonderful and mysterious individual, and it works perfectly for measuring the progress both in and out of the office. The problem is that, with our unique walking patterns and the limited space, it's common for the pedometer to undercount no matter how well known and reputable the brand-named pedometer is. At any rate, it's good that the pedometer always slants toward the low side. A couple of extra steps aren't going to hurt you, and when you inflate the conversion factor involved in the conversion from steps to calories, the manipulation will make some of the numerical differences go away.

I know this is a placebo effect, but it surely gave me a great sense of accomplishment and encouraged me to continue my daily exercise routine. I am a firm believer that errors within a complicated calculation will cancel each other out and make the final results accurate (in a relative sense). This mind-and-body connection thing really works.

Occasionally, if you've exercised beyond your limits, your knees and legs might become sore. That would be a great time to sit and take a water break and think about it carefully. After all, the point of exercising is to exercise your body as opposed to exhausting it. Knee is one of those body parts that cannot be naturally repaired once damaged. For people with a damaged knee, there is a legitimate excuse to procrastinate fitness training and sitting in a comfortable chair all day. But how will those patients eventually restart this process of revitalization and re-energizing in hope of getting healthy again?

One nifty trick to avoid knee pain is taking small steps and keeping your knees slightly bent in a natural position. This posture will shift a majority of the weight onto your thigh muscles, which are much sturdier than your knees. After a day's worth of walking and standing, there could be some part of your legs feeling sore and tired. If it is thigh and groin, that would be a badge of honor for your workout. If it is feet and heels, that would be OK, but you should probably rest more often. If it is inside your knee, and not the muscle surrounding it that hurts, then you should slow down to review and adjust the way you walk and stand.

STANDING

We've already talked about stand-up desks, so let's bring ourselves to the live subjects--standing human beings.

The important thing about standing, especially for long periods of time, is to make sure you're balanced and keep some movement shifting body weight around. Without this, certain muscles or joints will become stiff and sore fairly quickly. When standing, the first thing you should figure out is how to smoothly and constantly switch positions to exercise different groups of leg muscles. Although standing doesn't require as much energy as walking or running, it'll help cut down with belly fat as well as reducing the pressure on your spine.

Standing can also help reduce stress and the associated occupational hazards related to it. It's simple physics that when you sit, the middle part of your body forms many wrinkles. Whether these wrinkles going inward or outward, there will be stress. Yours truly once contracted a stomach ulcer from the stress of climbing the "corporate ladder" by sitting too much and typing out too many Word documents. That unpleasant experienced showed me the dangers of sitting and self-inflicted stress. Now at an older and wiser age without as much career ambitions as a young rookie, the hanging pressure cooker is taken out of the abdominal area. Everything just feels so much cooler, when working in the office these days.

(Standing up is an outstanding start.)

There's a lot of evidence supporting the idea that standing, even without moving around, can be more beneficial than sitting. Slightly shifting your center of gravity constantly to balance the stress applied to the various parts of your feet help you regain some agility of youth, although maintaining your center of balance is important throughout, so you don't hurt yourself. You can keep balance by shifting your weight the same way it naturally shifts during walks, thus mimicking a walking motion. You might be going nowhere, but it works. Standing still makes it more likely your feet will start hurting within a few days, and that will help to identify some pressure points at the bottom of your feet. After that, try to shift your weight about every half a minute and find a position that makes you comfortable. Then you will be able to stand several hours a day without hurting.

If you function on strict military-style instructions, you can keep your center of balance and shift your weight along your foot by alternating the foot you put your weight on every five or ten seconds. If all else fails, you can try walking in place; if you do that, keep your steps small. In addition to keeping yourself and by extension the body parts you're exercising more stable, remember that long steps can be more accident-prone to imitate while standing. When shifting around center of gravity, don't accidentally stretch something or get injured by going too fast or spanning out too wide. If you feel very uncomfortable or tired, sit down on your "office bench" and take a breather.

When people mention "typing", they're generally referring to the entire process involved with typing-- the planning beforehand, the rereading afterwards, and the wording throughout. Without properly doing the above three, it's hard to guarantee the quality of the work. Pivoting exercises are useful for the "befores" and "afters" of typing--they can be done in a cramped space and are much more simple and thoughtless than Tai Chi or walking patterns. Remember to pivot slowly and alternate the direction you're spinning in, so you don't get dizzy. Alternating the pivoting leg is as good as alternating directions in preventing dizziness.

In addition to the above mentioned, there are a lot of other stances you can exercise in. Since you're doing this while working in an office setting, go easily and pick non-demanding tasks, shifting slowly without causing a lot of noise or commotion. I've drawn some poses you can try out below.

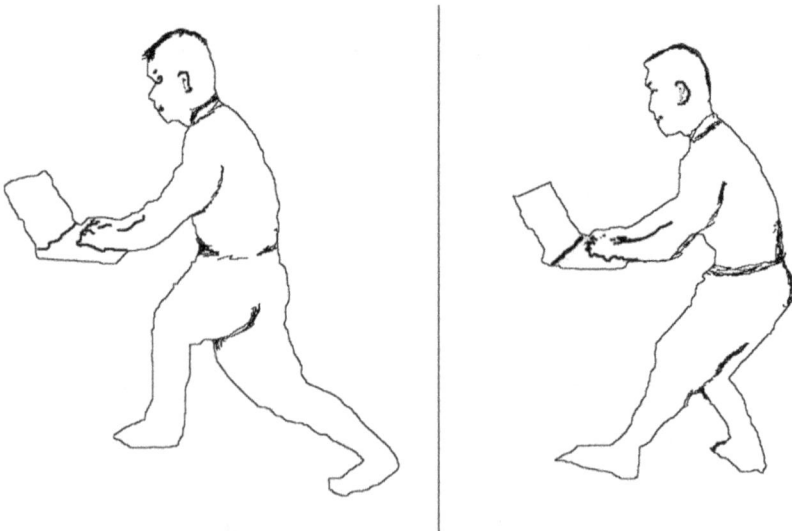

(Two poses that I've used most often.)

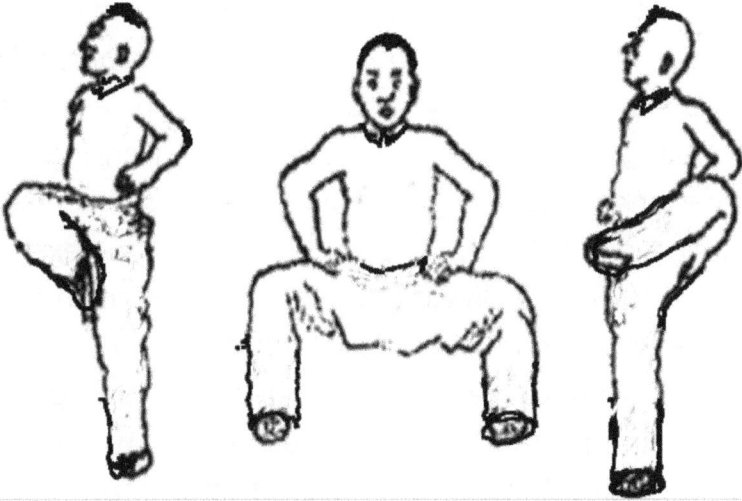

(Believe or not, I have tried these poses occasionally, but with hands on keyboard instead.)

When you're doing these exercises, try counting to about ten or twenty while breathing evenly in each stance. This is something akin to yoga, so focus on keeping your tension and relaxation simultaneously in one balancing act.

When you first start changing the way you work and adapting workout methods during your shift, you might find yourself tired at the end of each work day. If you start getting drowsy while driving home, drink a bit of coffee before leaving and try scaling down the next time you work out at work. It's a good idea to make sure you're making gradual lifestyle changes so you can drive safely and not overexerting yourself. Slow and steady really does win the race, after all. Start small and amp up slowly, and you should be able to sleep as comfortably after any decent workout afterwards.

When it comes to this, "patience" is the key to your exercise. The point of workout isn't to endanger your daily commute. You don't have to go from zero to sixty in one day. As long as you keep at it and change your lifestyle one day at a time, you'll eventually achieve a healthy weight. Yes, pushups and sit-ups are exercises targeted towards individual health. Without patience and perseverance, however, none of those will actually make anyone truly healthier. Patience is a virtue and gradual changes are more effective in the long run than sudden, rapid changes. The best way to start off is simply to stand more and sit less every day. Afterwards, you can start incorporating walking; as your body adapts, you'll be able to do more. The important thing is to know when to pause, take a breather, and start moving forward once more.

BELT

Most fitness gurus would tell you that belly fat is the hardest kind of fat to get rid of. Generally speaking, you need to burn a lot of calories before the belly fat starts to melt away; it can take a lot of exercise to even start making a dent in that belly, after you have bulging muscles in other areas.

There's a myth that goes around on the internet (yes, it's a myth) that NASA spent millions of dollars on a pointless venture to create pens that could write in zero gravity while the Soviet Union simply advised their astronauts to use pencils. While debate of the authenticity of the story is going on, the moral of the story still stands that simplicity is associated with practicality, low cost, low budget and winning. The words of von Clausewitz and KISS principle apply yet again--war is simple, yet "the simplest thing is difficult."

In the case of fitness, I'm referring to the tightening of your belt around a belly. What stops you from doing so? Nothing, really. There is, in fact, a surgery called "lap band" surgery that's basically a glorified, more expensive and stylish version of belt tightening. I have some co-workers who are off-chart with their BMI number, detected when attending an employer and insurance company sponsored free health care screening/consultation. And the advice they got from their visits to doctors are? Lap-band surgeries!

The operation is officially called "adjustable gastric band" surgery and when you look at the diagram that illustrates the procedure, it looks something like this:

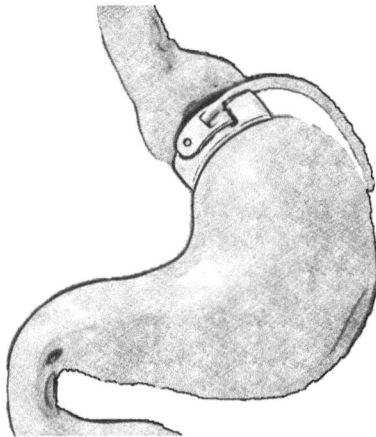

(An adjustable belt around the stomach in naked fashion)

It is a procedure that tightens a belt around the stomach inside the body. In reality, the same can be done outside the body with a normal belt as well. By tightening the belt several layers out, you can achieve the same results and avoid surgery, provided getting done early enough. It has in essence the same effects--the pressure on your digestive organs and the reduced appetite. If you get overly uncomfortable, try some of the deep breathing techniques we've mentioned in other paragraphs and drink some water. Thinking of this picture can also help, for that matter. After drinking some water while you take those deep breaths, if you start belching then you can be sure your rate of metabolism is changing, as you've learned in the chemistry lessons about equilibrium. Don't be too haste in tighten your belt, going up too many notches at one time, because you want this belt tightening to be still sufferable, at least more sufferable than having a real surgery. Again, think about that picture...

There's a different surgery called liposuction, but you should be even less tempted to try that one at home.

Fortunately, before your BMI got totally out of control, trying the simplified version of lap-band surgery is actually quite easy and could reverse the trend of your slipping down towards that expensive surgery. When you are hungry, the stomach acids inside your body will try to act out on you from within, as if trying to carve out your inner wall tissues and snatch nutrition from them. Such metabolic erosions are normal, and it happens when you are trying to lose weight just like you are in a state of hunger.

For some strange reason, a belt tightening around your waist, as long as you don't suffocate yourself and make it too difficult to breathe, will help slow down the secretion process of the stomach acid. Belt tightening has been quite a common practice in the third world countries when people were feeling hungry. The practice was used to make people feel better with a reduced appetite, imitating a state when the stomach is full with no empty spaces to take in more food. Sadly in poor countries, the cost of perennial belt-tightening is malnutrition for people, because of shortage of food and energy supplies. For overweight people with too much body fat, energy supply is not a problem. How to properly convert those fat into readily usable energy, and in a timely fashion, is the real challenge.

It's quite an annoyance for most office workers that body fat just stubbornly sits there and doesn't want to be converted into some forms of energy that make us healthy and active. The sad truth about getting rid of excessive calories is that certain heartburn and painful, fasting like sensation will need to be experienced one way or the other. Weight loss let you suffer through the same biological process as food shortage does. Well for me, that is a reminder to register fair amount of regrets for some gluttonous indulgences in some earlier days of my career. I felt thankful that I don't have to concern about malnutrition at least, and can count my blessings.

For belt tightening, I bought myself a special kind of belt that I can freely drill holes on.

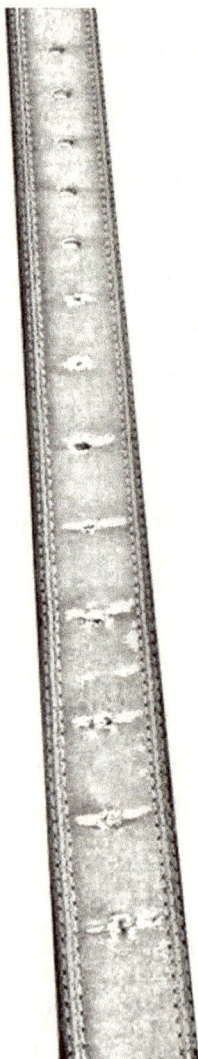

(DIY weight-loss belt, drills and drill bits not depicted)

You can also of course, buy the belts that have pre-made holes from beginning to the end like these.

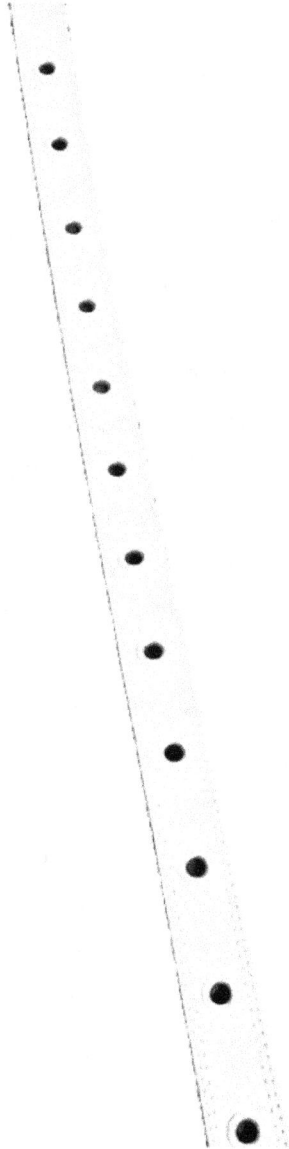

(Pre-drilled weight-loss belt)

For me, drilling new holes into the belt helps me see the progress I've made. Whether it's drilling a hole or moving yourself another notch up, you can take pride in the exercise you've done. Getting a shrinking belly is too important an historical event to be left without some form of recording.

Belt-tightening will effectively lead to some quite unexpected life changing consequences that one should be prepared for. These changes are related to increased metabolism and physiological reactions, and as we all know, biology can sometimes be a gross and nasty subject. At the beginning, it is possible the practice of tightening belt and walking more, will make one starts to perspire more. Secondly, with increasing amount of drinking water consumed, you might feel like passing gas more quickly and needing to use restrooms more often. These changes are all normal and logical. While thinking "Oh who am I kidding?" "Am I sure that I want to travel down this stinking path?" keep on carrying out your plans. Over the long run, it is all for a good cause, and yes, even for your co-workers. I would just try to pay extra attention to taking care of my business quietly. After a while, new routines are formed, new equilibriums would be reached, and nobody including you would notice anything unusual is going on.

When you have to clean yourself, you just have to get a relief and clean yourself. It is your responsibility to diligently keep yourself pollution free, so you can continue to get support from your neighbors. More frequent trips to the restroom also bring more opportunities to walk. After all, if you want that body you've got 20 years ago, you should be prepared to walk a "long, long" way to get there. Every bit of walk helps. It's the cumulative effect of many walks which will eventually lead to visible and significant changes in your body type.

During my many walking trips in the office, I started to reflect the fact that: 20 plus years ago, I joined the workforce and got a desk job. Gradually, every time I sit down, I felt that belly was pressing harder and harder against my belt. So I committed the cardinal sin, which was to relax this belt in my middle section just to be able to sit down a little more comfortably without feeling squeezed. I kept on giving myself excuse after excuse that I was reducing work related stress. Now look at these wonderful love handles of a Michelin tire spokesperson. In order to reverse that process, I would have to do the exact opposite; whenever I felt my belt was too loose, I tightened it a notch. It takes a while, yes; but combined with exercise and patience (there's that word again), I'm paying off the debt slowly. It takes many years to build up a big belly, after all; it's impractical to expect that one can get rid of it with a snap.

The patience we are talking about here is: not to endure the extreme amount of discomfort associated with grinding out of that excess fat, because too much pain and stress in stomach might break some other body parts. We are recommending small amount of discomfort applied slowly to the belly that is far away from the threshold of "suffering while evils are still sufferable". For many office professionals, it takes many years of seniority, marriages and years of having multiple children to get those big beer bellies. Envision tightening belt back to where it was at college graduation days in one squeeze, something catastrophic would be bound to happen. In fact, the practical thing to do is to tighten one notch, about half an inch to one inch, every three to six month. It is a good idea to ease back into good o days without squeezing the big o body too hard into other kinds of health breakdown.

If it takes more than six months to move one notch, so be it. Eight months a notch is still a notch as long as you don't go backward. And whenever you sit down for a break and feeling like it's too tight, it's okay to move back a notch and relax. It's okay to tell yourself you've had enough walking and standing for a day, if you truly had enough. It's still nice to relax once in a while even when you are in a weight watch program.

Remember that "be water" quote from Bruce Lee? That kind of thinking is the center around which this book revolves. Relaxation is healthy; once you've set your goal, you can be flexible as long as you know where you're going. You know the general direction of your plan, and if putting your nose to the grindstone ten times doesn't get there, do it a hundred times. If that doesn't work, try a thousand.

SUBPLOT

BREATHING, DRINKING, EATING, AND SUPPLEMENTAL EXERCISES

BREATHING

Breathing is a tool you can use, both on its own and alongside other exercises, to grind, melt or burn out excessive fat. Breathing can be done in a variety of ways, even though it is very rare for people to think about it consciously. We breathe continuously throughout our lives and won't live very long if breathing is somehow stopped for more than a minute. Considering how pervasive the activity called "breathing" is through everyone's life, the amount of training about breathing offered in formal school education system is disproportionally low. After formal schooling, for people who are aspired to become athletes, practice martial arts or learn yoga, it seems the topic of breathing would be mentioned more often in their trainings. Singers, teachers or salesmen might also receive trainings on breathing after entering the workforce, but not many other types of office employees could be so lucky. Whether from the office environment or from a gym, one common technique we want to emphasize here is to: learn to breathe with belly rather than chest, or breathe with diaphragm and stomach rather than lung.

Even though this kind of training is, for the most part, all about not breathing with "lung", but the ultimate goal of the technique is for increasing the "lung" capacity. Apparently, belly seems to be getting a bad deal here. We train our "belly" hard, and work our "belly" even harder, all for the benefits of other body parts like "lung" and "heart". That's just the way it is. We are favoring "lung capacity" here and are desperately trying to shrink that "belly capacity" so to speak. It's all part of the master plan to get healthy, so we can do more exercises to get even healthier.

These kinds of "breathing-with-stomach" technique used by salesmen, teachers, and singers is also one of the basic techniques that must be mastered by fitness enthusiasts who want to become so called "chi" masters.

There have been people posting questions to me about whether the "chi" exercise means the same thing as "chi" in "Tai Chi"? The answer is "No". "Chi" and "chi" could be written the same way in English, and are usually pronounced the same in English, but were written and pronounced differently in Chinese as two different words. In some movies about oriental martial arts, "chi" are often portrayed as this mystical thing with amazing feats of power. Even though "chi" can be literarily translated into the word "air" as in "airplane" or "air Jordan", flying and gliding around is not the ultimate goal for you to conduct the exercises and experiments with "chi". The reason to learn to control, maneuver or channel "chi" or "air" from one part of your body to another, is to learn to use the air outside of the body to help organize the air inside. For some strange reasons, but once pointed out it seems obvious, only air can be used to push air around within our bodies. No sharp or obtuse objects would be able to do the trick.

Like we've stated before, certain professions quite literally thrive on the way air moves through the body. Even if you're not a part of that work-field, learn the basic technique of using air to apply pressure to different parts of your body will help coordinate body movements and increase metabolism effectively.

The most basic breathing exercises aren't that interesting. Some people tried to make it fun by putting small objects (like coins) on their bellies and bouncing them up in the air, then watch them fall. Try it yourself and see how high you can get the coins to jump. For every set, try to repeat it five or ten times. Don't be too impatient with this exercise however; it's rare, but some people have gotten internal bleeding for addicting to this exercise too much. Believe it or not, either trying too hard or trying for too long with this exercise could be harmful.

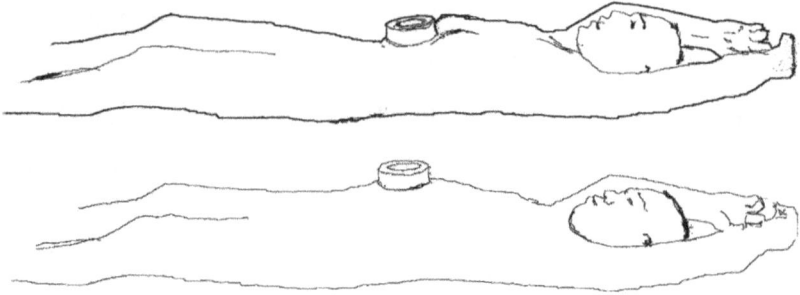

(I wasn't sure whether I have drawn the leg too long,
or the coin too big)

After repeating this exercise for a while, you can try using this motion (at a less erratic rate) in your everyday life, coordinating the stomach motion with your speaking, singing, pulling and pushing, walking, running, everything. You'll have learned to move "chi" around. Congratulations, you've become an entry level "chi" master.

...And that's about as far as we'll go into the practice of "chi". The function of "chi" has been widely disputed. Some believe it has supernatural powers and others simply label it as useless mumbo jumbo. No matter what, though, the same rules we've been enforcing apply; if you start feeling pain, stop exercising, rest, and tone it down next time. Keep going slowly; after all, "practice makes perfect" (even if what you're perfecting is monotonous and repetitive).

After practicing how to flex your belly while breathing, you can mimic that belly breathing at a slower and less sporadic pace throughout the day, and without lying down of course. Oh, by the way, you're now probably able to talk longer and therefore improve public speaking. You also might be a better teacher / trainer who doesn't need to pause as much during your speeches. You *also* could potentially become a better singer if you tried, but you really shouldn't do this in the office. The professional singers have their designated areas to push their air waves around.

Most important for us, however, the breathing practice will be just used to exercise and combat obesity. You might not be able to beat any Kung Fu masters, it's true, but you'll at least have learned how to use your abdominal muscle to accelerate your digestive process and increase your metabolism.

The long term effect of breathing exercises is the ability to increase your lung capacity dramatically and turn your belly into a powerful v6 engine that will propel you into a Marathon race without feeling tired. Well, if you don't reach that level, at the very least you'll be able to breathe easier.

In addition to this, exercising your breathing can also help you coordinate your motions and help you maintain a better balance with center of gravity in your body. Usually, the center of gravity for each of us happens to be slightly below, but aligned perfectly with the bellybutton. When you push, shove, jump or even hurdle over something, if your get your strength to originate from center of your gravity, you will be at your strongest and be least likely to get hurt. That is the benefit of breathing exercise in coordination with motions – to maintain good balance and be forceful. Exercising without balance is like driving a car without good alignment; one side will wear out faster than the other and eventually the entire machine breaks down.

Over the long run, the ability to breathe deeply will also help you with stress levels and help you become more calm and stoic. In essence, it helps you seem more "cool ".

Drinking

An overabundance of stomach acid can lead to diseases like stomach ulcers. I once had an ulcer; the doctor told me mine was in general attributable to stress and skipped lunches. The easiest way to deal with this is quite simple, however; simply drinking water to dilute the acid. Most of the beverages are typically surgery to be tasty, therefore are acidic to a certain level, making them less than ideal candidates to dilute acids. To solve the problem of stomach acid, the best thing for you to drink is water. Good news, water has "0" calories! No matter thinking about acidic drinks named "0" or sugary drinks not named after "0" as in calories, water is still the winner.

Admittedly, water can be tasteless and plain. The secret to getting over that is to make yourself thirsty. If you move and fidget around as much as you can in the office all day, you should be thirsty. If walking and standing by your desk isn't enough, I am going to say something not so popular here: "try to overload yourself with work my friend". Now we are seriously talking about using work to help you work out.

Try to plan your day well and make your schedule stuffed with tasks way more than you could handle. Then focus on every task intensely as if the fate of you and your employer depend on the outcome of it. Get your tasks finished as fast as you can with great anxiety and enthusiasm, even if you have to pretend. When you run around in the office, or run to the restroom, try not to get stopped and chat for too long along the way. Quip rather than BS when talking to people. If the above behavioral changes still do not get you thirsty, volunteer for the challenging tasks you usually won't take on. Alternatively, pick up a new skill that is deemed too fast-paced for your age. You'll get thirsty in no time. Being well hydrated is not easy. For folks exercising all day in the office, becoming energized, crazy and thirsty is quite easy.

When you feel like you are crazy and thirsty, plain water will finally become sweet.

Fortunately, the old standard of drinking eight "glasses of water" daily isn't an absolute must. I myself can very rarely finish eight glasses of water on any given day. Even with my new regiment of standing and walking (four to six hours a day), I just drink enough water to feel comfortable. When drinking, it's best to drink in small gulps and let the air out of stomach and acids diluted.

When drinking water to counter heartburn, small gulps help one trying to burp and preferably without making any detectable sounds. If you don't belch immediately after seeping, but still feel the hunger or the acid attacks inside you, try the breathing exercise described earlier. Fairly soon, you would feel all the air and void spaces inside your body getting shuffled around swapping places with water. Then bubbles will rise.

Office can be a cruel place sometimes, so it is worth emphasizing, when you burp, if you burp loudly, you will soon become the laughing stock of the entire office and then the entire planet, so take extra care not to disturb anybody else.

Drinking could be good no matter what time of the day it is, no, we are not talking about alcohol or soft drinks, but plain o' water. Timing of eating, on the other hand is an entirely different matter. It won't be equally good to eat just any time of the day, and there's something to be said about eating too late. If you want to eat a big meal, it is better to eat it in the morning, or afternoon but not at or after dinner time. If you eat in the earlier parts of the day, you would have plenty of time to digest what you have taken in, and even wash them away with water later.

If the last meal of your day is a stuffy one, and you still feel stuffed when going to bed, most likely the excessive food will accumulate in your body and turn into, you guessed it, belly fat. Therefore the best gauge for how full you are at dinner time is to ask yourself if you still have strong enough craving of your favorite food and do you still have space for some more. Then contrary to your urge, you should stop eating right there. The best time to leave dinner table is when you still want to eat, but no longer feel hungry. That way you will not get anorexia while still knowing you've got enough nutrients to be healthy.

But how do you get through the trying time before sleeping when you realized that you've miscalculated your appetite and truly ate too little at dinner? When you still want to eat something but can't, because you are up there with your daily rations, remember you have more flexibility in drinking than eating. Drink some water to dilute the stomach acids as you would during the day, or drink some milk if you still suffer and are truly miserable. Then next night, up your ration a little bit but not too much.

EATING

I eat when I'm hungry and stop when I don't feel hungry anymore; it's that simple. The word "feel" here is a relative word, of course; it's important to exercise caution with the word and make sure you're not overindulging.

With this philosophy (+ diligent daily workout), I get to enjoy eating anything I like and taste them like a judge in a cooking show. I don't have a taboo list for my diet. I do have a list of favorite food, but I won't stick to them in every meal. This is a free country, everyone is free to eat potato and steak every day. As long as we remember to eat with a small amount, even those food will not cause obesity. One gram of beef or potato each day, then stop eating completely is not going to get people overweight, but sounds rather like allocated amount in a survival training. Limiting the amount of food intake is more important in losing weight than restricting by variety, it's just simple physics, chemistry, or physiology, well, simple common sense really. In the name of "getting healthy" we should not go overboard with limiting amount of food either, because that can starve people to other problems if done to an extreme.

Moderation and balance is what this book's about. When long term food intake should be limited, we advocate cutting down the total amount of intake gradually. If one feels dizzy, faint or any other discomfort, then it's OK to take one step backward before moving two steps forward. Consult doctors and nutritionists while dieting.

When changing lifestyle, discomfort could be coming from various sources. I once find out my uncomfortable pains were coming from dehydration, like cramp, rather than a lack of food. I knew I still had enough energy supply, since I was heavy. But some muscle groups in the leg started feeling sore after I started to limit my meal size at lunch time. It turned out that I was not drinking enough fluid and not taking in enough salt. Just to show you that all those "low salt" advice on diet, when taking to an extreme could be harmful too.

Unless you're a nutritionist on the side, it's difficult to eye-measure the amount of calories in a dish just by looking at the plate of food. In everyday life, one should try to estimate a rough moderate and stick around that area. Try to remember a good plate of food that works for you and visualize in your brain the equivalent amount of food on the table compared to what you prefer. It's a crude estimation but it works well enough. For me, I stop eating when there's still space in my stomach for belt-tightening. If your BMI is too high, remember you still need to tighten your belt a notch. If you are already within your healthy BMI range, especially are at the low-end, you don't need to think about the next notch; focus on leaving enough space to take one deep breath without feeling a stomach explosions coming from the bellybutton. Then walk a little after eating.

As long as you mind the food intake and watch your waist size, there's no need to go on a very strict vegetarian diet. In general, a balanced diet is preferable over an unbalanced one. Even though most nutrients can be found in vegetables, and same thing cannot be said about meat, there are certain blends of vegetables that can get stuck in the intestines and slow down the digestive process. Intestinal obstructions that require surgery can be caused by pure vegetarian diets, in the same way plumbing pipes need minimum amount of lubrication. Too much of a good thing can be bad too.

Remember, we want to grind your belly into a thinner one over time as opposed to carving a smaller one within ten days. You don't have to treat eating like a chore, a race, a medical procedure, or a step-by-step task.

Eating regularly is a healthy habit, but if you have already had snacks excessively between meals then don't eat when the regular meal time arrives. Calculating the amount of calories you eat and picking a diet and exercise plan can be hard, but are essential for your health. You can either plan to eat regularly and resist all calls from office mates announcing "food in the kitchen", or you eat many small meals a day, and forget about the concept of "main course". The key is watching how much you've eaten and deciding how much you'll eat next. Be on alert for surpluses in food, as those can go south fast. Whether to go "breakfast"-"lunch"-"dinner" or "brunch"-"dinner"-"snack"-"snack" or five times of "snacks" all depend on the "+"s and "−"s with your calorie intake.

When you are overweight, try to skip a meal or two won't kill you or even make you sick of malnutrition. If anything, skipping a meal or two will even make you rejuvenated as long as you drink plenty of water and make common sense decisions, i.e. don't enter a contest to pull a bus or an 18 wheeler.

After skipping a few meals, don't forget to still eat like a judge in a cooking show. If you feast on two or three meals at once after skipping one meal, all your suffering from skipping meals have just gone for naught. Don't forget to tighten your belt and experience living with hunger a little bit. Now we are talking about a spiritual experience, with shortage of food. At least you will have plenty of safe and sanitized water to drink, then you can meditate and be thankful, thinking about all the people in this world who are still living in poverty.

Another ideological change came to mind after thanking God. This change is the attitude towards food left on the table. There was a time when throwing away food was a crime comparable to sneaking out of the house on a school night, back when I lived in the developing world.

Momma always said it's a sin or crime, at least shameful, to throw away food, therefore I should finish the dish instead of throwing away the excess into the dumpster. Well, that was then and this is now. When there were food shortage all around me, and everybody in the neighborhood seemed to be struggling to preserve food as much as possible for a rainy day, it was very inappropriate to waste food.

Nowadays living in the developed world where there are ample food everywhere, it is easy to commit a more heinous and sinister crime when we are stuffed up, but still see food left in the dishes. That crime is to throw away food into one's own stomach.

So what exactly have I done by throwing unneeded food into my stomach? First off, I've wasted the food just as much as I would've if I'd thrown it into the trash. Second, I've made myself overweight and prone to many kinds of sickness, which will

1) Disappoint teammates that rely on me in the office when I call in sick;
2) Cost my employer pay for my sick days;
3) Unintentionally raise insurance and health care cost for the nation;
4) Jeopardize the national security by increasing the government deficit, not to mention all the political infighting caused by this.

With that said, it's easier to throw away leftover food you're not planning on eating. If you do plan on eating those, I'd try not to cook anything new to accompany that food. In this environment we are living in, it's a little sad (or a blessing?) but true, stuffing yourself is a worse problem than throwing food away. The most responsible course of action is to order less at restaurants and cook less at home before eating.

There are places where ordering small amount of food is impossible, like in Texas or some Texas styled restaurants. Also it could be for economic reasons, that you've ordered a combo package and got a small mountain of food. In these cases, try eating that food slowly or spreading it out over multiple meals.

Like in the "smoke quitting" story we've mentioned earlier, if you really need a mental note to remind you about the guilt of throwing away food, try to get yourself a piggybank somewhere, and deposit the equivalent amount of money to the amount of food you are preparing to throw away. Then cast away the food anyway. At the end of the year, you will be able to total how much money you have wasted during the year. See whether you would have enough money to buy a nice Christmas gift for some citizens in the third world countries or donate to local charities.

Come to think of it, who would have thought throwing away food is now becoming a healthy habit on a high moral ground?

I am not a doctor and haven't even played one on TV either. Therefore you are welcome to use Google to search, or discuss with multiple medical doctors and ask them about novel concepts that has been discussed here with regard to unconventional eating habits. Would it be unhealthy when you skip a couple of meals periodically, while you still have a higher than normal BMI value. When you get their answers, jot down and compare. You will be surprised to see how little side effects fasting could have on your health comparing to problems that could be brought up by obesity. Even for the sake of breathing easier, it is worth going on hunger strike once in a while to let hunger strike you with a punch or two. It's better to take those punches than having obesity strike you down chronically.

SUSPENSION TRAINING

After you have started tightening a belt around your belly for a while, and your belly has slimmed down a bit, looking around, you might notice that you're starting to develop a rather unusual experience of weight loss. Unlike your fellow workout mates, miracle happens to you. Your belly is losing fat faster than your other body parts. That will leave you in a very awkward shape. Your belly's smaller, it's true; but the rest of you might not be, and you might find yourself looking a bit like the picture below.

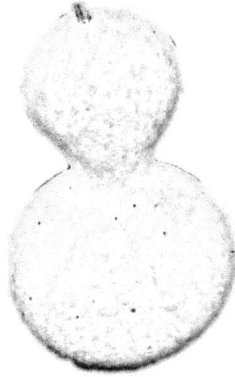

(It's not a *gourd* sign...get it? No? Okay.)

Naturally, this probably wasn't the shape you envisioned getting into when you started trying to lose weight. Trust me, as much as I like gourds, this isn't what the point of this book is either. So what do you do in this situation?

You shake things up a little.

I mean this in every way possible--literally, figuratively, statistically, physically, emotionally...er, well maybe not emotionally, but you get the picture. Suspend yourself from somewhere like a tree branch or something and pull your body upward. From there, shake out all your limbs. This isn't necessarily what you have to do by any stretch of the means, of course; the point of this is to get a full body exercise out of more muscle groups in you. Still, it couldn't hurt to start off with a tree or a doorframe.

Suspension training is useful for a decent amount of reasons. First off, your body weight is working against you. When you're suspended from (insert ceiling beam, doorframe, tree branch, etc), you're essentially taking a dumbbell the size of your own body weight into your hands and hoisting it upward. That's why pull-ups and chin-ups are absolutely energy efficient and environmental friendly in weight loss trainings. Heavier you are, a bigger weight you are pumping, that's the spirit!

The high bar (also known as the horizontal bar) is an Olympic gymnastics event. While everyone likes taking a look at that sort of event every once in a while, I don't think it's a good idea to try those moves of the Olympians at home. Not that many of us can perform those highfalutin moves anyway, and attempting it without experience can probably get yourself seriously injured. Unlike in parks or school yards, it is hard to find high bars in office buildings even in the office gyms, maybe employers don't want liabilities. You can generally find your standard set of monkey bars in the neighborhood parks, but they're often too short and busy (five year old traffic) to exercise from for long periods of time. It seems, they are becoming a less and less common piece of exercise equipment.

In my recollection, those "bar" equipment seemed to have an immunization effect to obesity. Human curiosity often makes us tactile creatures. When I was young, we had high bars in our playground, and kids would often get the urge to grab onto them during recesses just to "hang around". This sort of activity eventually led to some of the less athletic kids exercising a bit more with equipment like monkey bars alongside the high bars.

Office workers are a bit different though. As a child, you can adapt quickly and bounce back easily. As older people, our bodies are renewed at a much slower pace. Just because you were athletic as a child doesn't necessarily mean you'll be fit as an adult. For middle-aged office workers, it's harder if not impossible to recover after one hard exercise session. In addition, there aren't any adult-sized monkey bars; it is, as we've discussed, hard to find equipment outside the playground. Even in gymnasiums, most of the equipment is made for building muscle in your arms and legs and not for cutting fat in your waist by suspension. It would be nice if HR departments in different corporations can start to notice the exclusion principle between "bar" equipment and overweight population, and help to furnish office gyms differently. While waiting, it is worth shopping around to find gyms with good suspension equipment as supplemental exercise for your office routine.

While suspension can deal with belly fat quite quickly, there are a lot of people out there who can't do a single chin up yet (you're not alone) let alone sets of a dozen each time. Since simply dangling can only go so far, there are ways to ease yourself into that first chin up by starting with half of one.

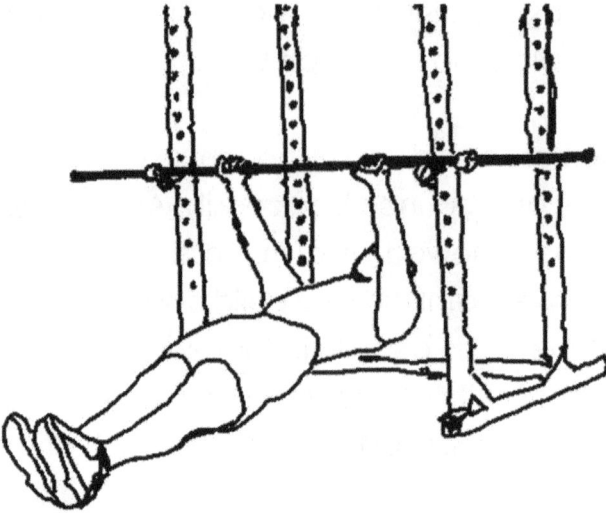

(Possibilities of doing ½, ¼ of a chin up, who said there's no math and science in sports?)

Once you can do multiple half chin ups, try doing a full one. After you can successfully do one, try two. Then three. Then four. After you've gotten to a dozen (cue hallelujah chorus), you can start on the next step--one handed chin ups.

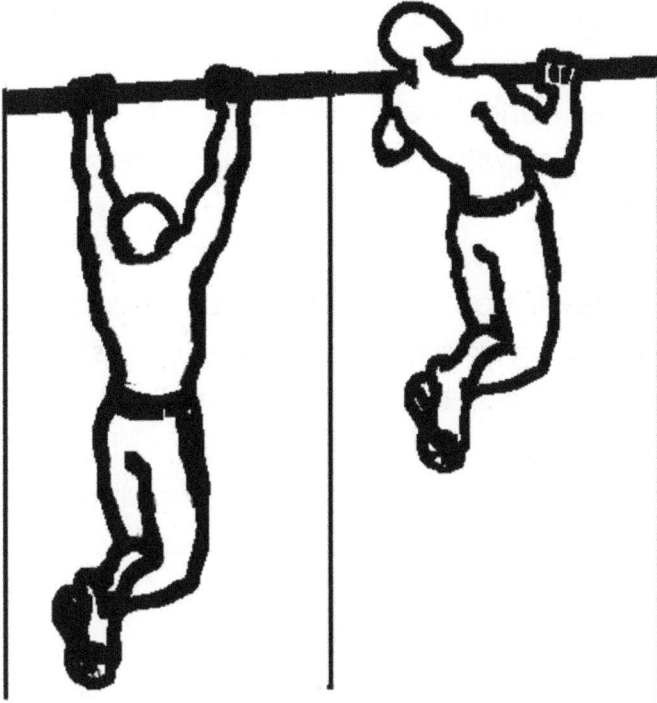

(Doing chin up with one hand is for advanced "bar" patrons.)

When you get to the level that you can safely utilize the bar with one hand, stop experimenting. We want you to have a healthy BMI, not try for the Olympics and possibly get injured. Know when to stop and why. An injury can wipe out all your fitness gains and set you far apart from being healthy and happy.

Hey, remember monkey bars? Finding those (for adults) are even harder than finding high bars. If you want to simulate that sort of motion, try shifting from left to right on the single bar. Besides helping your belly, it also helps some of the muscle groups in your hands, arms and chest.

An easier version of this is simply releasing the bar with one hand, re-grabbing it, and then repeating the motion with the other hand. To challenge yourself, see how long you can hang on with just one hand and breathe evenly several times.

Even if you never reach the level of one-handed chin ups, often suspending yourself for a few seconds at a time with one hand, likely can be sufficient to get you within healthy BMI range. It's not quite as easy as they make it look in the movies. If you can grab the bar with either one of your hands for a few seconds and breathe easily, don't try to be a hero and grab another person or object with your other hand. All those scenes in Hollywood movies are difficult to reproduce in real life, when one protagonist could grab onto a falling human body symbolizing the entire humanity and pull it upward. Then again, if it was in the movies, they probably could use stuntmen, special equipment and special effects.

RUNNING

Much like everything else in life, there exists in weight loss, the great concepts such as: "event horizon", "critical mass" and "virtuous circle". Once you've achieved a certain level of fitness, you'll burn calories even faster if you continue. If you've got to this point, then take confidence in the fact that you're home free. At this point, it's time to start running for the goal.

When I say "run", I mean literally "run" (as in "run, Forrest, run!"). You will be trimming off fat as fast as Forrest casting off his foot cast. I mean, really--how many active marathon runners have you seen in a state of poor health? All that walking and standing increases lung capacity, after all; the whole point of this book, in fact, is to help you achieve the same sort of deep breathing techniques these runners have. When you can run for a relatively good amount of time at a respectable speed without getting or feeling hurt, chances are you're in pretty good shape.

To get to that state, though, you need to invest a fair amount of time jogging indoor or outdoor. The treadmill's a great tool for this because it can ramp up anybody's speed at a very comfortable pace. Take me, for instance. I started off at walking speed (4.0 mph for me) and walked for an hour. The next day, I tried "4.1 mph"; however, sustaining that speed for one hour was too difficult. So I started off a bit more easily--50 minutes of 4.0 and 10 minutes of 4.1. Eventually by tweaking those numbers bit by bit between 50 and 10, I was able to ramp up my speed with very fine granularity.

The ideal healthy state I had in mind was being able to finish a Marathon under 5 hours without seriously hurting any body parts. This is still drastically different from how Senator John Glenn's health condition was when he was sent into the earth orbit for the second time. He was 76, with news outlets reporting his body was in the state of a

26 year old. That's some ideal fitness state only somebody like him could have achieved!

Obviously not everyone can achieve that kind of state, especially when at the age of 76. On the other hand, being like 26 at the age of 66, 56, 46 or even 36 are quite good also. One can slow down the aging clock by doing one of the oldest forms of exercise, which is running. Running is in some ways only a different form of walking. In fact, in ancient Chinese, the same word was used to describe both actions. When one cannot run, or walk, he or she is starting to get old. It was believed the first body part to get old is one's leg. After that, stagnation, aging, deterioration and the dreaded ultimate demise, this is really pessimistic now, will start to drop in and visit, one after another.

However, while running can help slow the aging clock, it can also cause wear and tear if you take it to the extreme. Exercising too much without resting or sleeping will cause your health to deteriorate. Like in walking, there are a few similar tips to keep yourself safe; for example, run with smaller steps and try not to stretch your knees into unnatural positions. When you want to increase speed, which is proportional to rate of burning calorie, increase frequency of those small steps rather than take big strides, in order to protect the knee. When running or jogging, try to distribute load mainly to your thigh muscles and groin. Always remember, when your knee hurts, rest and adjust the way you run.

SLEEPING

The first time I went to a fitness class, the trainer told us how muscles grew and got replaced in the body. He told us that a sore muscle indicates you've killed a lot of muscle cells, and that rest is required to let your body replace the dead cells with better, stronger ones. When you're feeling pain, your mind is sending your body messages to repair the damaged body parts with reinforcements. It's how stronger muscles, tougher calluses, and healthier bodies are formed. Those messages are, in a nutshell, called the mind and body connection. No pain no gain. The body needs to suffer some sort of pain and soreness to stimulate the brain to send those important messages to the body. That's why we need to exercise to get fit.

After you've done you part of exercising, there is, however, a catch--your mind can't repair your body if you're not getting enough sleep. It's a bit like a car can't be properly repaired unless you put it in a garage and turn off the engine. It's possible, to a certain point, to change tires while the car is still moving. But that point generally stops at TV race tracks. Similarly, you can heal some wounds without sleep, but you need to get enough sleep for serious healing and to lose weight.

If you exercise a muscle to the point where you wear it out completely, you could cause irreparable damages. As such, it's probably a good thing to give yourself enough rest after you've finished exercising. Without it, you'll only get the "pain" without getting back the much deserved reward that is called the "gain". Resting until you're not sore gives your body plenty of time to get reinforcement by replacing the dead cells with new ones. A good combination of sleep and a balanced diet helps further this process. In addition, sleep itself can help you maintain a better body--as long as you're not eating excessively, sleep can help you rearrange your body shape.

In general, just being able to lie down and sleep is pleasant. It was said that bedtime is the best time to achieve tranquility, peace, balance and equilibrium. I don't exactly know what all those words mean, but whatever they mean, they sound good to me.

Because overweight people often get tired easily, they found themselves falling into sleep a lot in different places. After falling into sleep more and more easily, they tend to draw the connection between increased weight and increased sleep; essentially, they might believe sleep is the cause of weight gain. This is, in fact, a misconception. It all depends on the message your body gets before sleeping--if you're taking well-exercised, "sore" muscles to sleep, then it can be very beneficial. If you go to sleep with a full stomach, the body will find areas to accumulate the food. The new cells will pile up with fat of excessive calorie, instead of replacing older ones. The mind-to-body connection works. Those messages translated by RNA to produce protein based on DNA, are very scientific, and work like clockwork every time. For some strange reasons, it works especially well in the dark, when you are sleeping.

OUTCOME

Once, there was a debate in my office among our lunch buddies regarding GDP and how it measures productivity. It starts in a rather trivial fashion: Peter went to throw away his brown paper bag and Paul chastised him, telling him that if he left it on the table and let the janitor take care of it, he would have generated more GDP.

Peter questioned this conclusion, and asked why his inactivity would have been considered more productive. Paul attempted to explain: productivity is a mysterious thing. Since we can't add "5 pages of Word document" to "5 tons of steel"; in other words, we can't measure the different areas of society against each other," all products would have to be converted into monetary terms to sum up the productivity for a society. GDP is calculated by tracking the amount of transactions in a region.

From here, Paul went on to say that if this "janitor" is not just merely a person, but a contracting firm that recruits thousands of janitors, and hire teams of lawyers and secretaries to handle paperwork, then more GDP would have been created by the act of not throwing away an empty brown bag, but let a firm of thousands of employees to move that mystical bag into a trash can. That's how productivity works in the corporate world and in our society.

The moral of this story is that, God works in mysterious ways to make us being productive and provide for our families. I believe that working without sitting down for majority of the working days would make me more productive, but someone else might disagree. I also believe it would help the team around me to be more productive by sitting less and moving around more, and save all of us a tremendous amount of health care costs for the society as a whole. Again, some people might not think the same, while some others start to stand up with me.

But who's to say what type of employees are contributing more to the corporation and the community, the ones sitting in their chairs or the ones standing by their desks? Hmmm... I am actually not interested in that debate.

What it comes down to is that I can confidently say when my boss comes to me and asks whether I've created value for the shareholders, I would always smile at him with positive attitude and told him that my career goals were aligned exactly as that of the company. Then in his evaluation, I get praised for being an excellent and productive employee. I get paid. And, as the cherry on top of the cake, I get to go home with a flat belly. In a way, it's like a legal and morally satisfying version of robbing a bank.

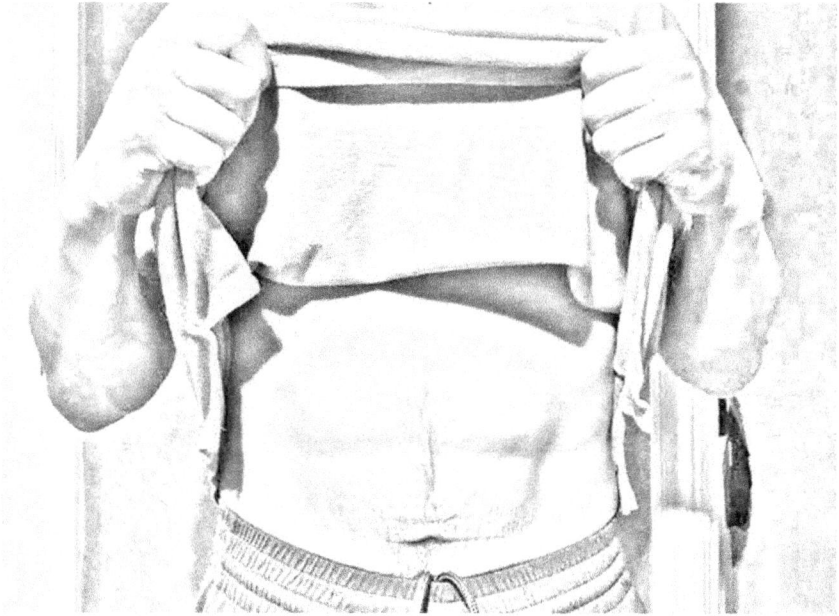

(At the end of the day)

The value of keeping a good "standing" in the company should never be underestimated, getting appreciated by immediate supervisor is priceless, but you ask me how much I have robbed from the bank? It's time for me to say "feeling like a million bucks". Sweet!

ABOUT THE AUTHORS

David Chen studied and worked in the areas of earth and environmental science during the earlier years of his career. He later shifted both his study and career interests to computer science and information technology, due to the growing popularity of the internet and markedly larger possibility of getting meaningful employment. His working years spent as a field geologist fostered his love for the great outdoors, and his software development and IT career gave birth to his passion for healthy working habits when working indoors. By a perfect blend of hyperactive enthusiasm in everything he sees outdoors, and a keen sense of amusement in everything he hears in the office, he was able to find the joy in healthy and happy living in everyday office work and can't wait to share it with the world.

Nora Mousas is a mythical creature that lives deep in the bowels of the internet. She enjoys writing and drawing but sadly is not proficient at either, although she is willing to try (hence participation in writing the book you are now holding). She also enjoys reading, which she luckily is proficient at.

www.ingramcontent.com/pod-product-compliance
Lightning Source LLC
Chambersburg PA
CBHW030026290326
41934CB00005B/503